THE PLANT REVOLUTION

Cruelty-free & Innovative Views
on Plants for Your Diet

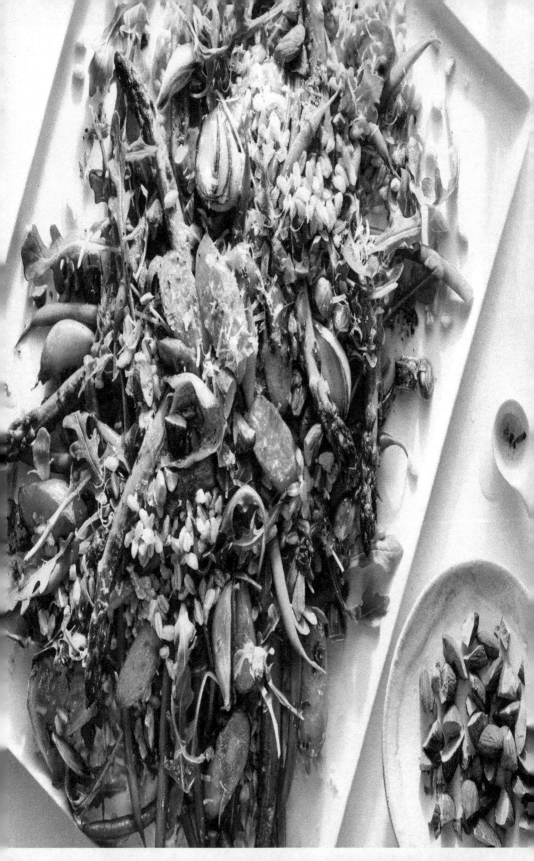

Table of Contents

INTRODUCTION

Eating healthy cannot be overemphasized in a world where fast food and junk food are always available. We all know that we could and should be eating healthier, but there are so many diets being advertised that it's hard to know what's best for you.

We're always reading about how processed foods are bad for your body. You may have also been advised repeatedly to avoid foods high in preservatives; however, no one likes to eat bland food or spend their time reading labels. This book will teach you how to find nutritious, delicious foods that will keep you satisfied while improving your health.

BENEFITS OF A BALANCED DIET

Before we dive into talking about the recipes and foods you need for a balanced diet, let's discuss a little more on the need for eating a balanced diet regularly.

- IMPROVED MEMORY: I know what you are thinking. "Are you being serious right now? If I just eat a few vegetables, I can be like Einstein?" Yes! You may not be as smart as Einstein, but healthy nutrients like Vitamins D, E, and C will help improve brain functionality.

- PREVENTS CANCER: According to medical experts, eating food that contains antioxidant can help protect cells from damage, thereby leading to a reduction in the risk of getting cancer. Cancer can also be treated at its early stage with healthy food.

- EMOTIONAL STABILITY: I know what you are thinking again. "Do you mean that if I'm going through a heartbreak and I eat some healthy food, I will be better?"

Yeah! It's not quite as straightforward as that, but healthy meals help improve your moods and balance your emotions. Scientists and researchers in 2016 found out that meals with a high glycemic load (high in carbohydrates) can trigger symptoms of depression and fatigue. Vegetables and fruits have a lower glycemic load and will help keep your blood sugar balanced.

- WEIGHT LOSS: Being overweight or obese can lead to other complicated illnesses like heart diseases, loss of bone density, and some types of cancer. Maintaining a healthful diet free from processed foods can help you stay at a healthy weight without resorting to fad diets.

- STRONG BONES AND TEETH: For healthy bones and teeth, a diet rich in calcium and magnesium is important. Maintaining bone integrity can reduce the risk of developing bone conditions later in life, such as osteoporosis.

Here are some foods that are rich in calcium:

- Low-fat dairy products
- Cabbage
- Legumes
- Broccoli
- Cauliflower
- Tofu

Now you know the awesome benefits of a healthy balanced diet, I'm sure you are on the edge of your seat waiting to see the healthy and easy-to-make meals planned out for you. Be sure to try them out and begin eating healthier today.
Enjoy!

BREAKFAST

Savory Spinach and Mushroom Crepes

Ready in about 120 minutes
Servings: 8
Per serving: Calories:680, Total Fat:71.8g, Saturated Fat:20.9g, Total Carbs:10g, Dietary Fiber:7g, Sugar:2g, Protein:3g, Sodium:525mg

Ingredients:
For the crepes:
- 6 cups rolled oats
- 2 tsps pink Himalayan salt
- 3 cups of soy milk
- 4 tbsps olive oil
- 2 tbsps almond butter
- 1 tsp nutmeg
- 4 tbsps egg replacement

For the filling:
- 2 lb. button mushrooms
- 20 oz fresh spinach, finely chopped
- 2 tbsps fresh rosemary, finely chopped
- 2 garlic cloves, crushed
- 4 tbsps olive oil
- 8 oz crumbled tofu
- 2 tbsps chia seeds

Directions:
- First, prepare the crepes. Combine all dry ingredients in a large bowl. Add milk, butter, nutmeg, olive oil, and egg replacement. Mix well

with a hand mixer at high speed. Transfer to a food processor and process until completely smooth.

- Grease a large nonstick pancake pan with some oil. Pour 1 cup of the mixture into the pan and cook for one minute on each side.
- Plug your instant pot and press the 'Sauté' button. Grease the stainless-steel insert with some oil and add mushrooms. Cook for 5 minutes, stirring constantly.
- Now add spinach, tofu, rosemary, and garlic. Continue to cook for another 5 minutes.
- Remove the mixture from the pot and stir in chia seeds. Let it sit for 10 minutes.
- Meanwhile, grease a small baking pan with some oil and line it with parchment paper.
- Divide the mushroom mixture between crepes and roll-up. Gently transfer to a prepared baking pan.
- Wrap the pan with aluminum foil and set it aside.
- Pour 1 cup of water into your instant pot and set the steam rack. Put the pan on top and seal the lid. Press the 'Manual' button and set the timer for 10 minutes.
- When done, release the pressure naturally, and open the lid.
- Optionally, sprinkle with some dried oregano before serving.

Tomato and Pesto Toast

Ready in about: 5 minutes

Servings: 8

Per serving: Calories: 214 Cal Fat: 7.2 g Carbs: 32 g Protein: 6.5 g Fiber: 3 g

Ingredients:

- 2 small tomatoes, sliced
- ½ teaspoon ground black pepper
- 2 tablespoons vegan pesto
- 4 tablespoons hummus
- 2 slices of whole-grain bread, toasted
- Hemp seeds as needed for garnishing

Directions:

- Spread hummus on one side of the toast, top with tomato slices and then drizzle with pesto.
- Sprinkle black pepper on the toast along with hemp seeds, and then serve straight away.

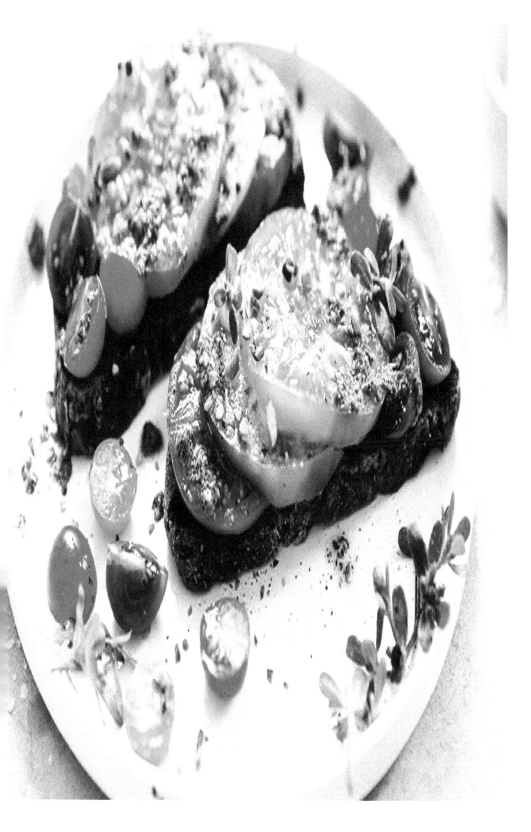

Mushroom Avocado Panini

Ready in about: 40 minutes

Servings: 8

Per serving: Calories 338 Fats 22. 4g Carbs 25. 5g Protein 12. 4g

Ingredients:

- 2 tbsps olive oil
- 2 cups sliced white button mushrooms
- Salt and black pepper to taste
- 2 ripe avocado, pitted, peeled, and sliced
- 4 tbsps freshly squeezed lemon juice
- 2 tbsps chopped parsley
- 1 tsp pure maple syrup
- 16 slices whole-wheat ciabatta
- 8 oz sliced plant-based Parmesan cheese
- 2 tbsps olive oil

Directions:

- Heat the olive oil in a medium skillet over medium heat and sauté the mushrooms until softened, 5 minutes. Season with salt and black pepper. Turn the heat off.
- Preheat a panini press to medium heat, 3 to 5 minutes.
- Mash the avocado in a medium bowl and mix in the lemon juice, parsley, and maple syrup.

- Spread the mixture on 4 bread slices, divide the mushrooms and plant-based Parmesan cheese on top.
- Cover with the other bread slices and brush the top with olive oil.
- Grill the sandwiches one after another in the heated press until golden brown, and the cheese melted.
- Serve warm.

Chocolate-Mango Quinoa Bowl

Ready in about: 35 minutes

Servings: 4

Ingredients

- 2 cups quinoa
- 2 tsps ground cinnamon
- 2 cups non-dairy milk
- 2 large mango, chopped
- 6 tbsps unsweetened cocoa powder
- 4 tbsps almond butter
- 2 tbsps hemp seeds
- 2 tbsps walnuts
- ½ cup raspberries

Directions

- In a pot, combine the quinoa, cinnamon, milk, and 1 cup of water over medium heat. Bring to a boil, low heat, and simmer covered for 25-30 minutes.

- In a bowl, mash the mango and mix cocoa powder, almond butter, and hemp seeds.

- In a serving bowl, place cooked quinoa and mango mixture. Top with walnuts and raspberries. Serve immediately.

Strawberry & Pecan Breakfast

Ready in about: 15 minutes

Servings: 4

Ingredients

- 2 (14-oz) can coconut milk, refrigerated overnight
- 2 cups granola
- 1 cup pecans, chopped
- 2 cups sliced strawberries

Directions

- Drain the coconut milk liquid. Layer the coconut milk solids, granola, and strawberries in small glasses. Top with chopped pecans and serve right away.

- Enjoy!

Cashew Cheese Pimiento Biscuits

Ready in about: 30 minutes
Servings: 8
Ingredients

- 4 cups whole-wheat flour
- 4 tsps baking powder
- 2 tsps salt
- 1 tsp baking soda
- 1 tsp garlic powder
- ½ tsp black pepper
- 1/2 cup plant butter, cold and cubed
- 1 cup coconut milk
- 2 cups shredded cashew cheese
- 2 (4 oz) jar chopped pimientos,
- 2 tbsps melted unsalted plant butter

Directions

- Preheat the oven to 450 F and line a baking sheet with parchment paper. Set aside. In a medium bowl, mix the flour, baking powder, salt, baking soda, garlic powder, and black pepper. Add the cold butter using a hand mixer until the mixture is the size of small peas. Pour in ¾ of the coconut milk and continue whisking. Continue adding the remaining coconut milk, a tablespoonful at a time, until dough forms.

- Mix in the cashew cheese and pimientos. (If the dough is too wet to handle, mix in a little bit more flour until it is manageable). Place the dough on a lightly floured surface and flatten the dough into ½-inch thickness.

- Use a 2 ½-inch round cutter to cut out biscuits' pieces from the dough. Gather, re-roll the dough once and continue cutting out biscuits. Arrange the biscuits on the prepared pan and brush the tops with the melted butter. Bake for 12-14 minutes, or until the biscuits are golden brown. Cool and serve.

- Enjoy!!

Ciabatta Bread Pudding with Sultanas

Ready in about: 2 hours 10 minutes
Servings: 8
Per serving: Calories: 458; Fat: 10.4g; Carbs: 81.3g; Protein: 11.4g

Ingredients

- 4 cups coconut milk, unsweetened
- 1 cup agave syrup
- 2 tablespoons coconut oil
- 1 teaspoon vanilla essence
- 1 teaspoon ground cardamom
- 1/2 teaspoon ground cloves
- 1 teaspoon ground cinnamon
- 1/2 teaspoon Himalayan salt
- 3/2 pounds stale ciabatta bread, cubed
- 1/2 cup sultana raisins

Directions

- In a mixing bowl, combine the coconut milk, agave syrup, coconut oil, vanilla, cardamom, ground cloves, cinnamon, and Himalayan salt.
- Add the bread cubes to the custard mixture and stir to combine well. Fold in the sultana raisins and allow it to rest for about 1 hour on a counter.
- Then, spoon the mixture into a lightly oiled casserole dish.

- Bake in the preheated oven at 350 degrees F for about 1 hour or until the top is golden brown.
- Place the bread pudding on a wire rack for 10 minutes before slicing and serving. Bon appétit!

Raspberry and Chia Smoothie Bowl

Ready in about: 10 minutes
Servings: 4
Per serving: Calories: 442; Fat: 10.9g; Carbs: 85g; Protein: 9.6g

Ingredients

- 2 cups coconut milk
- 4 small-sized bananas, peeled
- 3 cups raspberries, fresh or frozen
- 4 dates, pitted
- 2 tablespoons coconut flakes
- 2 tablespoons pepitas
- 4 tablespoons chia seeds

Directions

- In your blender or food processor, mix the coconut milk with the bananas, raspberries, and dates.
- Process until creamy and smooth. Divide the smoothie between two bowls.
- Top each smoothie bowl with coconut flakes, pepitas, and chia seeds. Bon appétit!

Mixed Berry and Almond Butter Swirl Bowl

Ready in about:10 minutes
Servings: 6
Per serving: Calories: 397; Fat: 16.3g; Carbs: 48.5g; Protein: 19.6g

Ingredients

- 3 cups almond milk
- 4 small bananas
- 4 cups mixed berries, fresh or frozen
- 6 dates, pitted
- 6 scoops hemp protein powder
- 6 tablespoons smooth almond butter
- 4 tablespoons pepitas

Directions

- In your blender or food processor, mix the almond milk with the bananas, berries, and dates.
- Process until everything is well combined. Divide the smoothie between three bowls.
- Top each smoothie bowl with almond butter and use a butter knife to swirl the almond butter into the top of each smoothie bowl.
- Afterwards, garnish each smoothie bowl with pepitas, serve well-chilled and enjoy!

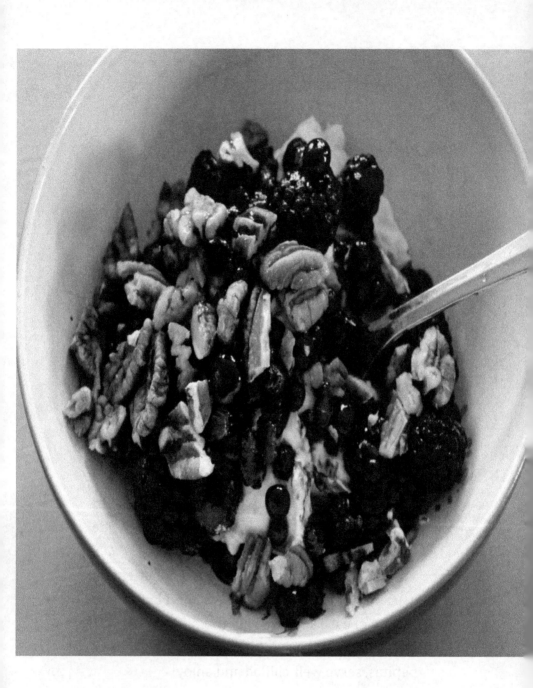

The Best Chocolate Granola Ever

Ready in about: 1 hour
Servings: 20)
Per serving: Calories: 428; Fat: 23.4g; Carbs: 46.4g; Protein: 11.3g

Ingredients

- 1 cup coconut oil
- 1 cup agave syrup
- 2 teaspoons vanilla paste
- 6 cups rolled oats
- 1 cup hazelnuts, chopped
- 1 cup pumpkin seeds
- 1 teaspoon ground cardamom
- 2 teaspoons ground cinnamon
- 1/2 teaspoon ground cloves
- 2 teaspoons Himalayan salt
- 1 cup dark chocolate, cut into chunks

Directions

- Begin by preheating your oven to 260 degrees F; line two rimmed baking sheets with a piece of parchment paper.
- Then, thoroughly combine the coconut oil, agave syrup, and vanilla in a mixing bowl.
- Gradually add in the oats, hazelnuts, pumpkin seeds, and spices; toss to coat well. Spread the mixture out onto the prepared baking sheets.

- Bake in the middle of the oven, stirring halfway through the cooking time, for about 1 hour or until golden brown. Stir in the dark chocolate and let your granola cool completely before storing. Store in an airtight container.
- Bon appétit!

LUNCH

Classic Garlicky Rice

Ready in about: 20 minutes
Servings: 8
Per serving: Calories: 422; Fat: 15.1g; Carbs: 61.1g; Protein: 9.3g

Ingredients

- 8 tablespoons olive oil
- 8 cloves of garlic, chopped
- 3 cups white rice
- 5 cups vegetable broth

Directions

- In a saucepan, heat the olive oil over a moderately high flame. Add in the garlic and sauté for about 1 minute or until aromatic.
- Add in the rice and broth. Bring to a boil; immediately turn the heat to a gentle simmer.
- Cook for about 15 minutes or until all the liquid has been absorbed. Fluff the rice with a fork, season with salt and pepper, and serve hot!
- Enjoy!

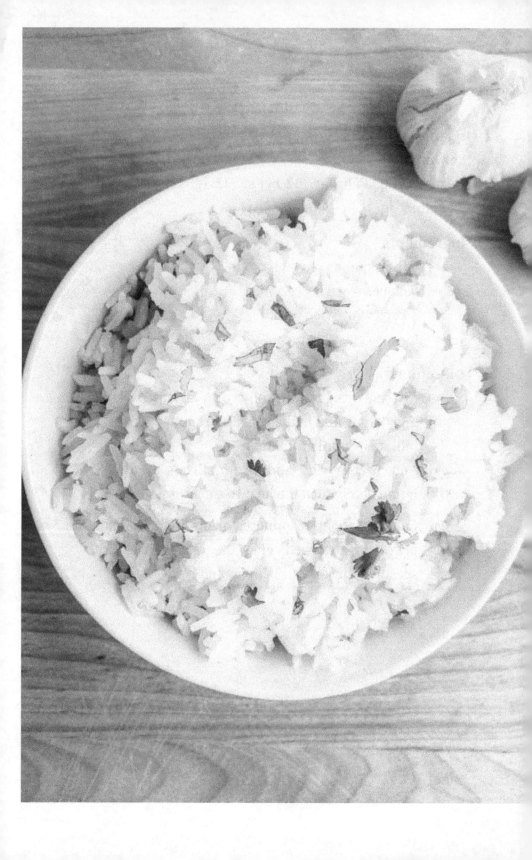

Country Cornbread with Spinach

Ready in about: 50 minutes
Servings: 8
Per serving: Calories: 282; Fat: 15.4g; Carbs: 30g; Protein: 4.6g

Ingredients

- 2 tablespoons flaxseed meal
- 2 cups all-purpose flour
- 2 cups yellow cornmeal
- 1 teaspoon baking soda
- 1 teaspoon baking powder
- 2 teaspoons kosher salt
- 2 teaspoons brown sugar
- A pinch of grated nutmeg
- 1 1/2 cup oat milk, unsweetened
- 2 teaspoons white vinegar
- 1 cup olive oil
- 4 cups spinach, torn into pieces

Directions

- Start by preheating your oven to 420 degrees F. Now, spritz a baking pan with a nonstick cooking spray.
- To make the flax eggs, mix flaxseed meal with 3 tablespoons of water. Stir and let it sit for about 15 minutes.

- In a mixing bowl, thoroughly combine the flour, cornmeal, baking soda, baking powder, salt, sugar, and grated nutmeg.
- Gradually add in the flax egg, oat milk, vinegar, and olive oil, constantly whisking to avoid lumps. Afterwards, fold in the spinach.
- Scrape the batter into the prepared baking pan. Bake your cornbread for about 25 minutes or until a tester inserted in the middle comes out dry and clean.
- Let it stand for about 10 minutes before slicing and serving.
- Bon appétit!

Creamy Spinach Artichoke Pasta

Ready in about: 15 minutes

Servings: 4

Per serving: Calories 457, Total Fat 36. 2g, Saturated Fat 29. 6g, Cholesterol 40mg, Sodium 779mg, Total Carbohydrate 27. 6g, Dietary Fiber 4g, Total Sugars 4. 7g, Protein 10. 3g

Ingredients:

- 2 tablespoons butter
- 1/2 teaspoon garlic powder
- 2 cups vegetable broth
- 2 cups of coconut milk
- 1/2 teaspoon salt
- Freshly cracked pepper
- 1 cup pasta
- 1/2 cup fresh baby spinach
- 1 cup quartered artichoke hearts
- 1/4 cup grated Parmesan cheese

Directions:

- In the Instant Pot, hit "Sauté," add butter when it melts, add garlic powder just until it's tender and fragrant.
- Add the vegetable broth, coconut milk, salt, some freshly cracked pepper, and pasta. Place the lid on the pot and lock it into place to seal. Pressure

Cook on High Pressure for 4 minutes. Use Quick Pressure Release.

- Add the spinach, a handful at a time, to the hot pasta and toss it in the pasta until it wilts into Instant Pot in Sauté mode. Stir the chopped artichoke hearts into the pasta. Sprinkle grated Parmesan over the pasta, then stir slightly to incorporate the Parmesan. Top with an additional Parmesan, then serve.

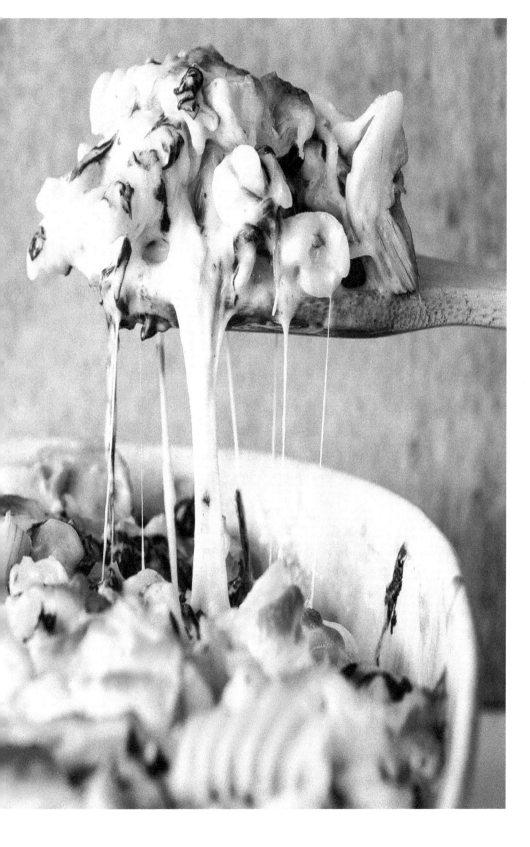

Cheese Beetroot Greens Macaroni

Ready in about: 15 minutes
Servings: 4
Per serving: Calories 147, Total Fat 8g, Saturated Fat 4. 8g, Cholesterol 23mg, Sodium 590mg, Total Carbohydrate 12. 7g, Dietary Fiber 1g, Total Sugars 1. 5g, Protein 6. 5g

Ingredients:
- 2 tablespoons butter
- 2 cloves of garlic minced
- 2 cups button mushrooms
- 1 bunch beetroot greens
- 1 cup vegetable broth
- 1 cup macaroni
- 1/2 teaspoon salt
- 1 cup grated Parmesan cheese
- Freshly cracked pepper

Directions:
- In the Instant Pot, hit "Sauté," add butter, garlic and slice the mushrooms. Add the beetroot greens to the pot along with 1/2 cup vegetable broth. Stir the beetroot greens as it cooks until it is fully wilted.

- Add vegetable broth, macaroni, salt, and pepper. Place lid on Instant Pot and lock into place to seal. Pressure Cook on High Pressure for 4 minutes. Use Quick Pressure Release. Add grated Parmesan cheese.

Fresh Tomato Mint Pasta

Ready in about: 15 minutes

Servings: 4

Per serving: Calories 350, Total Fat 18. 5g, Saturated Fat 14. 3g, Cholesterol 54mg, Sodium 47mg, Total Carbohydrate 39. 4g, Dietary Fiber 1. 9g, Total Sugars 2g, Protein 8. 7g

Ingredients:

- 2 cups of pasta
- 2 tablespoons coconut oil
- 1 teaspoon garlic powder
- 2 tomatoes
- 1 tablespoon butter
- 1/2 cup fresh mint
- 1/2 cup of coconut milk
- Salt & pepper to taste
- Enough water

Directions:

- Add the coconut oil to the Instant Pot, hit "Sauté," add in the garlic, and stir. Add the tomatoes and a pinch of salt. Then add mint and pepper.
- Next, add coconut milk, butter, and water. Stir well; lastly, add in the pasta.
- Secure the lid and hit "Keep Warm/Cancel" and then hit "Manual" or "Pressure Cook" High Pressure for 6 minutes. Quick-release when done.
- Enjoy.

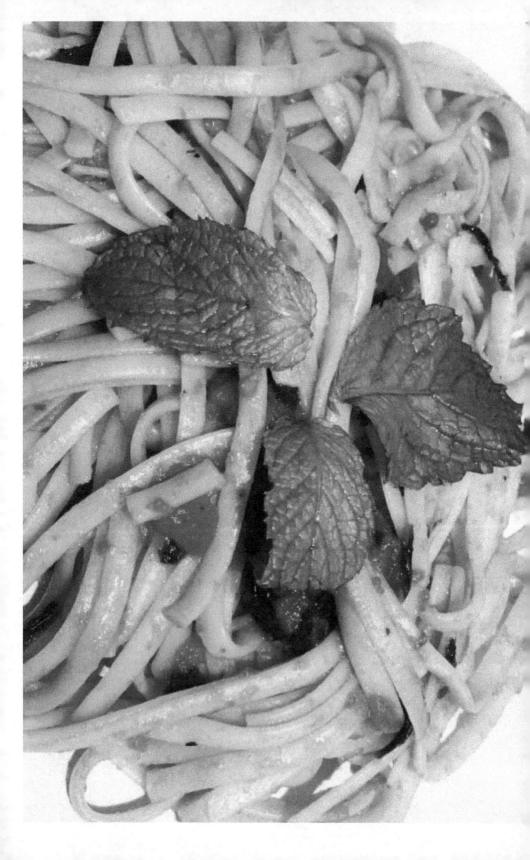

Pasta with Eggplant Sauce

Ready in about: 15 minutes

Servings: 4

Per serving: Calories 306, Total Fat 18g, Saturated Fat 12. 9g, Cholesterol 30mg, Sodium 188mg, Total Carbohydrate 27g, Dietary Fiber 12. 6g 45%, Total Sugars 13. 9g, Protein 14. 2g

Ingredients:

- 2 tablespoons coconut oil
- 4 cloves of garlic
- 2 small onions
- 2 medium eggplants
- 2 cups diced tomatoes
- 2 tablespoons tomato sauce
- 1/2 teaspoon dried thyme
- 1 teaspoon honey
- Pinch paprika
- Freshly cracked pepper
- 1/2 salt and pepper, or to taste
- 12 oz. spaghetti
- 4 cups vegetable broth
- Handful fresh coriander, chopped

Directions:

- Set Instant Pot to Sauté. Add the coconut oil and allow it to melt. Add the onion and garlic and cook for 2 minutes or until the onion is soft and transparent.

- Add eggplant, diced tomatoes, tomato sauce, thyme, honey, paprika, and freshly cracked pepper. Stir them well to combine; add spaghetti, and vegetable broth, salt, and pepper.
- Lock the lid and make sure the vent is closed. Set Instant Pot to Manual or Pressure Cook on High Pressure for 10 minutes. When cooking time ends, release pressure and wait for steam to completely stop before opening the lid.
- Top each serving with grated goat and a sprinkle of fresh coriander.

Spicy Veggie Steaks with Green Salad

Ready in about: 35 minutes
Servings: 4
Ingredients

- 2 eggplant, sliced
- 2 zucchinis, sliced
- 1/2 cup coconut oil
- Juice of a lemon
- 10 oz plant-based cheddar, cubed
- 20 Kalamata olives
- 4 tbsps pecans
- 2 oz mixed salad greens
- 1 cup tofu mayonnaise
- Salt to taste
- 1 tsp Cayenne pepper to taste

Directions

- Set oven to broil and line a baking sheet with parchment paper. Arrange eggplant and zucchini on the baking sheet. Brush with coconut oil and sprinkle with cayenne pepper. Broil for 15-20 minutes.

- Remove to a serving platter and drizzle with the lemon juice. Arrange the plant-based cheddar cheese, Kalamata olives, pecans, and mixed greens with the grilled veggies. Top with tofu mayonnaise and serve.

Tofu & Spinach Lasagna with Red Sauce

Ready in about: 65 minutes
Servings: 8
Ingredients

- 4 tbsps plant butter
- 2 white onions, chopped
- 2 garlic cloves, minced
- 5 cups crumbled tofu
- 6 tbsps tomato paste
- 1 tbsp dried oregano
- Salt and black pepper to taste
- 2 cups baby spinach
- 16 tbsps flax seed powder
- 3 cups cashew cream cheese
- 10 tbsps psyllium husk powder
- 4 cups coconut cream
- 10 oz grated plant-based mozzarella
- 4 oz grated plant-based Parmesan
- 1 cup fresh parsley, finely chopped

Directions

- Melt plant butter in a medium pot and sauté onion and garlic until fragrant and soft, about 3 minutes. Stir in tofu and cook until brown. Mix in tomato paste, oregano, salt, and black pepper. Pour ½ cup of water into the pot, stir, and simmer the ingredients until most of the liquid has evaporated.

- Preheat oven to 300 F. Mix flax seed powder with 1 ½ cups water in a bowl to make vegan "flax egg." Allow sitting to thicken for 5 minutes. Combine vegan "flax egg" with cashew cream cheese and salt. Add psyllium husk powder a bit at a time while whisking and allow the mixture to sit for a few minutes. Line a baking sheet with parchment paper and spread the mixture in. Cover with another parchment paper and flatten the dough into the sheet. Bake for 10-12 minutes. Slice the pasta into sheets.

- In a bowl, combine coconut cream and two-thirds of the plant-based mozzarella cheese. Fetch out 2 tablespoons of the mixture and reserve. Mix in plant-based Parmesan cheese, salt, pepper, and parsley. Set aside. Grease a baking dish with cooking spray, layer a single line of pasta, spread with some tomato sauce, 1/3 of the spinach, and ¼ of the coconut cream mixture. Repeat layering the ingredients twice in the same manner, making sure to top the final layer with the coconut cream mixture and the reserved cream cheese. Bake for 30 minutes at 400 F. Slice and serve with salad.

Avocado Coconut Pie

Ready in about: 80 minutes

Servings: 8

Ingredients

Piecrust:
- 2 tbsps flax seed powder + 3 tbsps water
- 2 cups coconut flour
- 8 tbsps chia seeds
- 2 tbsps psyllium husk powder
- 2 tsps baking soda
- 2 pinches salt
- 6 tbsps coconut oil
- 8 tbsps water

Filling:
- 4 ripe avocados, chopped
- 2 cups tofu mayonnaise
- 6 tbsps flax seed powder + 9 tbsps water
- 4 tbsps fresh parsley, chopped
- 2 jalapenos finely chopped
- 1 tsp onion powder
- 1/2 tsp salt
- 1 cup cream cheese
- 5/2 cup grated plant-based Parmesan

Directions

- In 2 separate bowls, mix the different portions of flax seed powder with the respective quantity of water. Allow absorbing for 5 minutes.

- Preheat oven to 350 F. In a food processor, add the piecrust ingredients and the smaller portion of the vegan "flax egg." Blend until the resulting dough forms into a ball. Line a springform pan with parchment paper and spread the dough in the pan. Bake for 10-15 minutes.

- Put the avocado in a bowl and add the tofu mayonnaise, remaining vegan "flax egg," parsley, jalapeno, onion powder, salt, cream cheese, and plant-based Parmesan. Combine well. Remove the piecrust when ready and fill with the creamy mixture. Bake for 35 minutes. Cool before slicing and serving.

Mushroom & Green Bean Biryani

Ready in about: 50 minutes
Servings: 8
Ingredients

- 2 cups of brown rice
- 6 tbsps plant butter
- 6 medium white onions, chopped
- 12 garlic cloves, minced
- 2 tsps ginger puree
- 2 tbsps turmeric powder + for dusting
- 1/2 tsp cinnamon powder
- 4 tsps garam masala
- 1 tsp cardamom powder
- 1 tsp cayenne powder
- 1 tsp cumin powder
- 2 tsps smoked paprika
- 6 large tomatoes, diced
- 4 green chilies, minced
- 2 tbsps tomato puree
- 2 cups chopped cremini mushrooms
- 2 cups chopped mustard greens
- 2 cups plant-based yogurt

Directions

- Melt the butter in a large pot and sauté the onions until softened, 3 minutes. Mix in the garlic, ginger, turmeric, cardamom powder, garam masala, cardamom powder, cayenne pepper, cumin powder, paprika, and salt. Stir-fry for 1-2 minutes.

- Stir in the tomatoes, green chili, tomato puree, and mushrooms. Once boiling, mix in the rice and cover it with water. Cover the pot and cook over medium heat until the liquid absorbs and the rice is tender, 15-20 minutes. Open the lid and fluff in the mustard greens and half of the parsley. Dish the food, top with the coconut yogurt, garnish with the remaining parsley, and serve warm.

DINNER

Kimchi Stew

Preparation Time: 35 minutes

Servings: 8

Per serving: Calories: 153 Cal Fat: 8.2 g Carbs: 25 g Protein: 8.4 g Fiber: 2.6 g

Ingredients:

- 2 pounds of tofu, extra-firm, pressed, cut into 1-inch pieces
- 8 cups napa cabbage kimchi, vegan, chopped
- 2 small white onions, peeled, diced
- 4 cups sliced shiitake mushroom caps
- 3 teaspoons minced garlic
- 4 tablespoons soy sauce
- 4 tablespoons olive oil, divided
- 8 cups vegetable broth
- 4 tablespoons chopped scallions

Directions:

- Take a large pot, place it over medium heat, add 1 tablespoon oil and when hot, add tofu pieces in a single layer and cook for 10 minutes until browned on all sides.
- When cooked, transfer tofu pieces to a plate, add remaining oil to the pot and when hot, add onion and cook for 5 minutes until soft.

- Stir in garlic, cook for 1 minute until fragrant, stir in kimchi, continue cooking for 2 minutes, then add mushrooms and pour in broth.
- Switch heat to medium-high level, bring the mixture to boil, then switch heat to medium-low level, and simmer for 10 minutes until mushrooms are softened.
- Stir in tofu, taste to adjust seasoning, and garnish with scallions.
- Serve straight away.

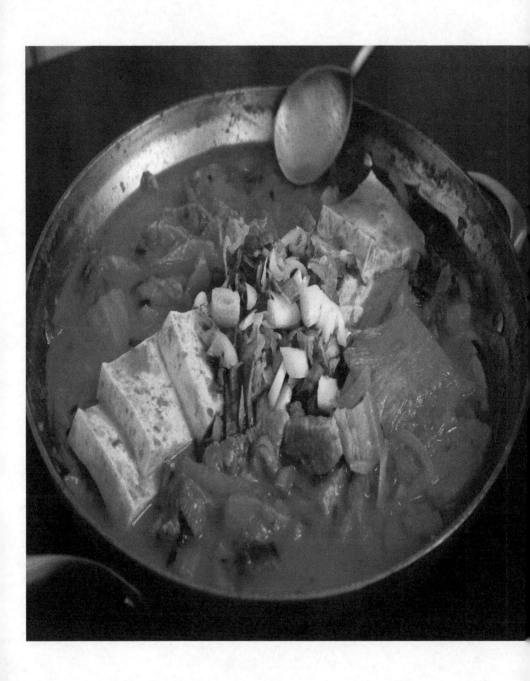

Spicy Bean Stew

Ready in about: 60 minutes

Servings: 8

Per serving: Calories: 114 Cal Fat: 1.6 g Carbs: 19 g Protein: 6 g Fiber: 8.4g

Ingredients:

- 14 ounces cooked black eye beans
- 28 ounces chopped tomatoes
- 4 medium carrots, peeled, diced
- 7 ounces cooked kidney beans
- 2 leeks, diced
- 1 chili, chopped
- 2 teaspoons minced garlic
- 1/6 teaspoon ground black pepper
- 1/3 teaspoon salt
- 2 teaspoons red chili powder
- 2 lemon, juiced
- 6 tablespoons white wine
- 2 tablespoons olive oil
- 5/6 cups vegetable stock

Directions:

- Take a large saucepan, place it over medium-high heat, add oil and when hot, add leeks and cook for 8 minutes or until softened.

- Then add carrots, continue cooking for 4 minutes, stir in chili and garlic, pour in the wine, and continue cooking for 2 minutes.
- Add tomatoes, stir in lemon juice, pour in the stock and bring the mixture to boil.
- Switch heat to medium level, simmer for 35 minutes until stew has thickened, then add both beans along with remaining ingredients and cook for 5 minutes until hot.
- Serve straight away.
- Enjoy!

Root Vegetable Stew

Ready in about: 8 hours and 10 minutes
Servings: 12
Per serving: Calories: 120 Cal Fat: 1 g Carbs: 28 g Protein: 4 g Fiber: 6 g

Ingredients:

- 4 cups chopped kale
- 2 large white onions, peeled, chopped
- 2-pounds of parsnips, peeled, chopped
- 2-pounds of potatoes, peeled, chopped
- 4 celery ribs, chopped
- 2-pounds butternut squash, peeled, deseeded, chopped
- 2-pounds carrots, peeled, chopped
- 6 teaspoons minced garlic
- 2-pounds sweet potatoes, peeled, chopped
- 2 bay leaves
- 2 teaspoons ground black pepper
- 1 teaspoon sea salt
- 2 tablespoons chopped sage
- 6 cups vegetable broth

Directions:

- Switch on the slow cooker, add all the ingredients in it, except for the kale, and stir until mixed.
- Shut the cooker with a lid and cook for 8 hours at a low heat setting until cooked.

- When done, add kale into the stew, stir until mixed, and cook for 10 minutes until leaves have wilted.
- Serve straight away.
- **Enjoy!**

Homemade Kitchari

Ready in about: 40 minutes

Servings: 10

Ingredients

- 8 cups chopped cauliflower and broccoli florets
- 1 cup split peas
- 1 cup brown rice
- 2 red onions, chopped
- 2 (14.5-oz) can diced tomatoes
- 6 garlic cloves, minced
- 2 jalapeño peppers, seeded
- 1 tsp ground ginger
- 2 tsps ground turmeric
- 2 tsps olive oil
- 2 tsps fennel seeds
- Juice of 2 large lemon
- Salt and black pepper to taste

Directions

- In a food processor, place the onion, tomatoes with juices, garlic, jalapeño pepper, ginger, turmeric, and 2 tbsps of water. Pulse until ingredients are evenly mixed.

- Heat the oil in a pot over medium heat. Cook the cumin and fennel seeds for 2-3 minutes, stirring often. Pour in the puréed mixture, split peas, rice, and 3 cups of water. Bring to a boil, then lower the heat and simmer for 10 minutes. Stir in cauliflower, broccoli, and cook for another 10 minutes. Mix in lemon juice and adjust seasoning.

Asian Quinoa Sauté

Ready in about: 30 minutes
Servings: 8
Ingredients

- 2 cups quinoa
- Salt to taste
- 2 heads of cauliflower, break into florets
- 4 tsps untoasted sesame oil
- 2 cups snow peas, cut in half
- 2 cups frozen peas
- 4 cups chopped Swiss chard
- 4 scallions, chopped
- 4 tbsps water
- 2 tsps toasted sesame oil
- 2 tbsps soy sauce
- 4 tbsps sesame seeds

Directions

- Place quinoa with 2 cups of water and salt in a bowl. Bring to a boil, lower the heat and simmer for 15 minutes. Do not stir.

- Heat the oil in a skillet over medium heat and sauté the cauliflower for 4-5 minutes. Add in snow peas and stir well. Stir in Swiss chard, scallions, and 2 tbsps of water; cook until wilted, about 5 minutes. Season with salt.

- Drizzle with sesame oil and soy sauce and cook for 1 minute. Divide the quinoa in bowls and top with the cauliflower mixture. Garnish with sesame seeds and soy sauce to serve.

Mediterranean-Style Lentil Salad

Ready in about: 20 minutes + chilling time
Servings: 10
Per serving: Calories: 348; Fat: 15g; Carbs: 41.6g; Protein: 15.8g

Ingredients

- 3 cups red lentil, rinsed
- 2 teaspoons deli mustard
- 1 lemon, freshly squeezed
- 4 tablespoons tamari sauce
- 4 scallion stalks, chopped
- ½ cup extra-virgin olive oil
- 4 garlic cloves, minced
- 2 cups butterhead lettuce, torn into pieces
- 4 tablespoons fresh parsley, chopped
- 4 tablespoons fresh cilantro, chopped
- 2 teaspoons fresh basil
- 2 teaspoons fresh oregano
- 3 cups cherry tomatoes, halved
- 6 ounces Kalamata olives, pitted and halved

Directions

- In a large-sized saucepan, bring 4 ½ cups of the water and the red lentils to a boil.
- Immediately turn the heat to a simmer and continue to cook your lentils for about 15 minutes or until tender. Drain and let it cool completely.

- Transfer the lentils to a salad bowl; toss the lentils with the remaining ingredients until well combined.
- Serve chilled or at room temperature.
- Bon appétit!

Creamed Green Bean Salad with Pine Nuts

Ready in about: 10 minutes + chilling time

Servings: 5

Per serving: Calories: 308; Fat: 26.2g; Carbs: 16.6g; Protein: 5.8g

Ingredients

- 3 pounds green beans, trimmed
- 4 medium tomatoes, diced
- 4 bell peppers, seeded and diced
- 8 tablespoons shallots, chopped
- 1cup pine nuts, roughly chopped
- 1 cup vegan mayonnaise
- 2 tablespoons deli mustard
- 4 tablespoons fresh basil, chopped
- 4 tablespoons fresh parsley, chopped
- 1 teaspoon red pepper flakes, crushed
- Sea salt and freshly ground black pepper, to taste

Directions

- Boil the green beans in a large saucepan of salted water until they are just tender or about 2 minutes.
- Drain and let the beans cool completely; then, transfer them to a salad bowl. Toss the beans with the remaining ingredients.
- Taste and adjust the seasonings.
- Bon appétit!

Hearty Cream of Mushroom Soup

Ready in about: 15 minutes
Servings: 10
Per serving: Calories: 308; Fat: 25.5g; Carbs: 11.8g;
Protein: 11.6g

Ingredients

- 4 tablespoons soy butter
- 2 large shallot, chopped
- 40 ounces Cremini mushrooms, sliced
- 4 cloves garlic, minced
- 8 tablespoons flaxseed meal
- 10 cups vegetable broth
- 4/6 cups full-fat coconut milk
- 2 bay leaf
- Sea salt and ground black pepper, to taste

Directions

- In a stockpot, melt the vegan butter over medium-high heat. Once hot, cook the shallot for about 3 minutes until tender and fragrant.
- Add in the mushrooms and garlic and continue cooking until the mushrooms have softened. Add in the flaxseed meal and continue to cook for 1 minute or so.
- Add in the remaining ingredients. Let it simmer, covered and continue to cook for 5 to 6 minutes more until your soup has thickened slightly.
- Bon appétit!

Quinoa and Black Bean Salad

Ready in about: 15 minutes + chilling time
Servings: 8
Per serving: Calories: 433; Fat: 17.3g; Carbs: 57g;
Protein: 15.1g

Ingredients

- 4 cups water
- 2 cups quinoa, rinsed
- 32 ounces canned black beans, drained
- 4 Roma tomatoes, sliced
- 2 red onions, thinly sliced
- 2 cucumbers, seeded and chopped
- 4 cloves garlic, pressed or minced
- 4 Italian peppers, seeded and sliced
- 4 tablespoons fresh parsley, chopped
- 4 tablespoons fresh cilantro, chopped
- 1/2 cup olive oil
- 2 lemons, freshly squeezed
- 2 tablespoons apple cider vinegar
- 1 teaspoon dried dill weed
- 1 teaspoon dried oregano
- Sea salt and ground black pepper, to taste

Directions

- Place the water and quinoa in a saucepan and bring it to a rolling boil. Immediately turn the heat to a simmer.

- Let it simmer for about 13 minutes until the quinoa has absorbed all of the water; fluff the quinoa with a fork and let it cool completely. Then, transfer the quinoa to a salad bowl.
- Add the remaining ingredients to the salad bowl and toss to combine well. Bon appétit!

Classic Roasted Pepper Salad

Ready in about: 15 minutes + chilling time
Servings: 6
Per serving: Calories: 178; Fat: 14.4g; Carbs: 11.8g;
Protein: 2.4g

Ingredients

- 12 bell peppers
- 6 tablespoons extra-virgin olive oil
- 6 teaspoons red wine vinegar
- 6 garlic cloves, finely chopped
- 4 tablespoons fresh parsley, chopped
- Sea salt and freshly cracked black pepper, to taste
- 1 teaspoon red pepper flakes
- 12 tablespoons pine nuts, roughly chopped

Directions

- Broil the peppers on a parchment-lined baking sheet for about 10 minutes, rotating the pan halfway through the cooking time until they are charred on all sides.
- Then, cover the peppers with plastic wrap to steam. Discard the skin, seeds, and cores.
- Slice the peppers into strips and toss them with the remaining ingredients. Place in your refrigerator until ready to serve. Bon appétit!

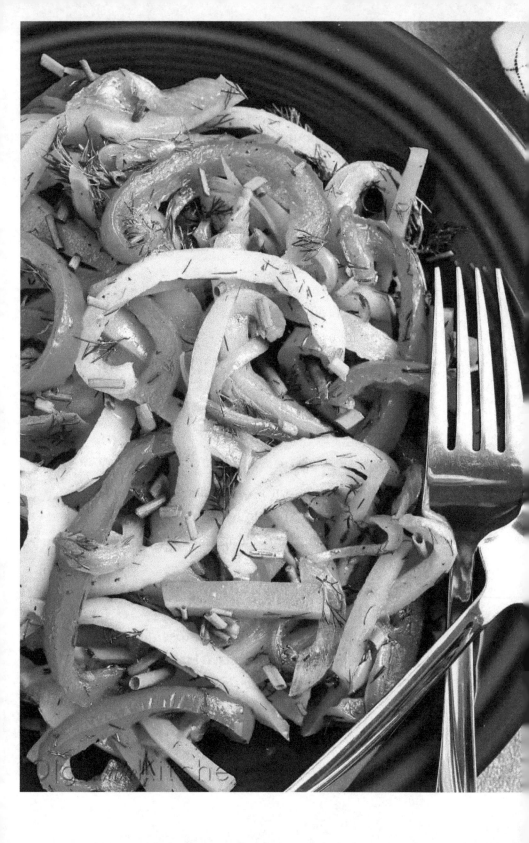

DESSERTS

Southern Apple Cobbler with Raspberries

Ready in about: 50 minutes

Servings: 8

Ingredients

- 6 apples, chopped
- 4 tbsps pure date sugar
- 2 cups fresh raspberries
- 4 tbsps unsalted plant butter
- 1 cup whole-wheat flour
- 2 cups toasted rolled oats
- 4 tbsps pure date sugar
- 2 tsps cinnamon powder

Directions

- Preheat the oven to 350 F and grease a baking dish with some plant butter.

- Add apples, date sugar, and 3 tbsps of water to a pot. Cook over low heat until the date sugar melts and then mix in the raspberries. Cook until the fruits soften, 10 minutes. Pour and spread the fruit mixture into the baking dish and set aside.

- In a blender, add the plant butter, flour, oats, date sugar, and cinnamon powder. Pulse a few times until crumbly. Spoon and spread the mixture on the fruit mix until evenly layered. Bake in the oven for 25 to 30 minutes or until golden brown on top. Remove the dessert, allow cooling for 2 minutes, and serve.

- Enjoy!

Baked Apples Filled with Nuts

Ready in about: 35 minutes + cooling time | Servings: 8

Ingredients

- 8 gala apples
- 6 tbsps pure maple syrup
- 8 tbsps almond flour
- 12 tbsps pure date sugar
- 12 tbsps plant butter, cold and cubed
- 2 cups chopped mixed nuts

Directions

- Preheat the oven the 400 F.

- Slice off the top of the apples and use a melon baller or spoon to scoop out the cores of the apples. In a bowl, mix the maple syrup, almond flour, date sugar, butter, and nuts. Spoon the mixture into the apples and then bake in the oven for 25 minutes or until the nuts are golden brown on top and the apples soft. Remove the apples from the oven, allow cooling, and serve.

- Enjoy!

Brownie Energy Bites

Ready in about: 1 hour and 10 minutes
Servings: 4
Per serving: Calories: 174.6 Cal Fat: 8.1 g Carbs: 25.5 g
Protein: 4.1 g Fiber: 4.4 g

Ingredients:
- 1 cup walnuts
- 2 cups Medjool dates, chopped
- 1 cup almonds
- 1/4 teaspoon salt
- 1 cup shredded coconut flakes
- 2/3 cup
- 4 teaspoons cocoa powder, unsweetened

Directions:
- Place almonds and walnuts in a food processor and pulse for 3 minutes until the dough starts to come together.
- Add remaining ingredients, reserving ¼ cup of coconut, and pulse for 2 minutes until incorporated.
- Shape the mixture into balls, roll them in remaining coconut until coated, and refrigerate for 1 hour.
- Serve straight away

Mango Coconut Cheesecake

Preparation Time: 4 hours and 10 minutes

Servings: 8

Per serving: Calories: 200 Cal Fat: 11 g Carbs: 22.5 g Protein: 2 g Fiber: 1 g

Ingredients:

For the Crust:

- 2 cups macadamia nuts
- 2 cups dates, pitted, soaked in hot water for 10 minutes

For the Filling:

- 4 cups cashews, soaked in warm water for 10 minutes
- 1 cup and 2 tablespoons maple syrup
- 2/3 cup and 4 tablespoons coconut oil
- 1/2 cup lemon juice
- 1 cup and 4 tablespoons coconut milk, unsweetened, chilled

For the Topping:

- 2 cups fresh mango slices

Directions:

- Prepare the crust, and for this, place nuts in a food processor and process until mixture resembles crumbs.

- Drain the dates, add them to the food processor and blend for 2 minutes until a thick mixture comes together.
- Take a 4-inch cheesecake pan, place date mixture in it, spread and press evenly, and set aside.
- Prepare the filling and for this, place all its ingredients in a food processor and blend for 3 minutes until smooth.
- Pour the filling into the crust, spread evenly, and then freeze for 4 hours until set.
- Top the cake with mango slices and then serve.
- **Enjoy!!**

Cookie Dough Bites

Ready in about: 4 hours and 10 minutes
Servings: 36
Per serving: Calories: 200 Cal Fat: 9 g Carbs: 26 g
Protein: 1 g Fiber: 0 g

Ingredients:
- 30 ounces cooked chickpeas
- 2/3 cup vegan chocolate chips
- 2/3 cup and 2 tablespoons peanut butter
- 16 Medjool dates pitted
- 2 teaspoons vanilla extract, unsweetened
- 4 tablespoons maple syrup
- 3 tablespoons almond milk, unsweetened

Directions:
- Place chickpeas in a food processor along with dates, butter, and vanilla and then process for 2 minutes until smooth.
- Add remaining ingredients, except for chocolate chips, and then pulse for 1 minute until blended and dough comes together.
- Add chocolate chips, stir until just mixed, then shape the mixture into 18 balls and refrigerate for 4 hours until firm.
- Serve straight away
- Enjoy!!

Date Cake Slices

Ready in about: 1 hour 40 minutes
Servings: 8
Per Serving: Calories 850 Fats 61. 2g Carbs 65. 7g
Protein 12. 8g

Ingredients:
- 1 cup cold plant butter, cut in pieces, plus extra for greasing
- 2 tbsps flax seed powder + 3 tbsps water
- 1 cup whole-wheat flour, plus extra for dusting
- ½ cup chopped pecans and walnuts
- 2 tsps baking powder
- 2 tsps baking soda
- 2 tsps cinnamon powder
- 2 tsps salt
- 2/3 cup water
- 2/3 cup pitted dates, chopped
- 1 cup pure date sugar
- 2 tsps vanilla extract
- ½ cup pure date syrup for drizzling.

Directions:
- Preheat the oven to 350 F and lightly grease a round baking dish with some plant butter.
- In a small bowl, mix the flax seed powder with water and allow thickening for 5 minutes to make the flax egg.

- In a food processor, add the flour, nuts, baking powder, baking soda, cinnamon powder, and salt. Blend until well combined.
- Add the water, dates, date sugar, and vanilla. Process until smooth with tiny pieces of dates evident.
- Pour the batter into the baking dish and bake in the oven for 1 hour and 10 minutes or until a toothpick inserted comes out clean. Remove the dish from the oven, invert the cake onto a serving platter to cool, drizzle with the date syrup, slice, and serve.
- **Enjoy!**

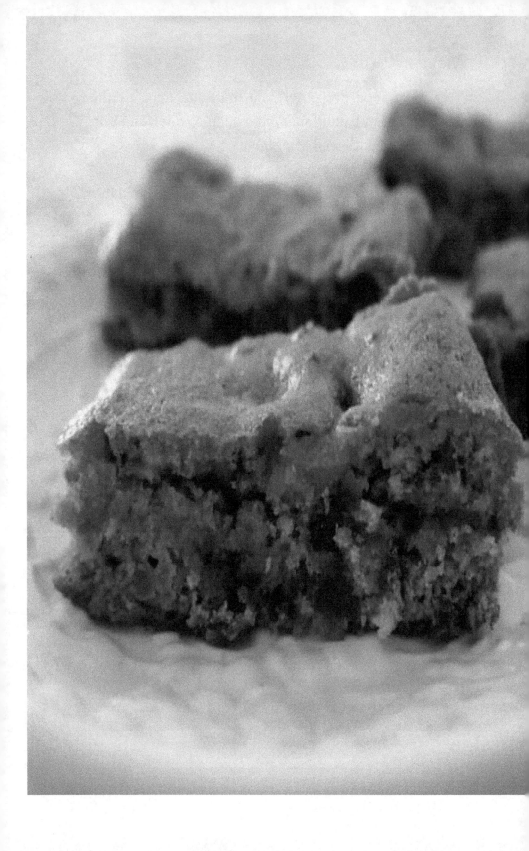

Muhammara Dip with a Twist

Ready in about: 35 minutes
Servings: 18
Per serving: Calories: 149; Fat: 11.5g; Carbs: 8.9g; Protein: 2.4g

Ingredients

- 6 red bell peppers
- 10 tablespoons olive oil
- 4 garlic cloves, chopped
- 2 tomatoes, chopped
- 3/2 cup bread crumbs
- 4 tablespoons molasses
- 2 teaspoons ground cumin
- 1/2 sunflower seeds, toasted
- 2 Maras pepper, minced
- 4 tablespoons tahini
- Sea salt and red pepper, to taste

Directions

- Start by preheating your oven to 400 degrees F.
- Place the peppers on a parchment-lined baking pan. Bake for about 30 minutes; peel the peppers and transfer them to your food processor.
- Meanwhile, heat 2 tablespoons of the olive oil in a frying pan over medium-high heat. Sauté the garlic and tomatoes for about 5 minutes or until they've softened.

- Add the sautéed vegetables to your food processor. Add in the remaining ingredients and process until creamy and smooth.
- Bon appétit!

Avocado with Tangy Ginger Dressing

Ready in about: 10 minutes
Servings: 8)
Per serving: Calories: 295; Fat: 28.2g; Carbs: 11.3g; Protein: 2.3g

Ingredients

- 4 avocados, pitted and halved
- 2 cloves of garlic, pressed
- 2 teaspoons fresh ginger, peeled and minced
- 2 tablespoons balsamic vinegar
- 8 tablespoons extra-virgin olive oil
- Kosher salt and ground black pepper, to taste

Directions

- Place the avocado halves on a serving platter.
- Mix the garlic, ginger, vinegar, olive oil, salt, and black pepper in a small bowl. Divide the sauce between the avocado halves.
- Bon appétit!

Easy Lebanese Toum

Ready in about: 10 minutes
Servings: 12
Per serving: Calories: 252; Fat: 27g; Carbs: 3.1g; Protein: 0.4g

Ingredients
- 4 heads garlic
- 2 teaspoons coarse sea salt
- 3 cups olive oil
- 2 lemons, freshly squeezed
- 4 cups carrots, cut into matchsticks

Directions
- Puree the garlic cloves and salt in your food processor of a high-speed blender until creamy and smooth, scraping down the sides of the bowl.
- Gradually and slowly, add in the olive oil and lemon juice, alternating between these two ingredients to create a fluffy sauce.
- Blend until the sauce has thickened. Serve with carrot sticks and enjoy!
- Enjoy!

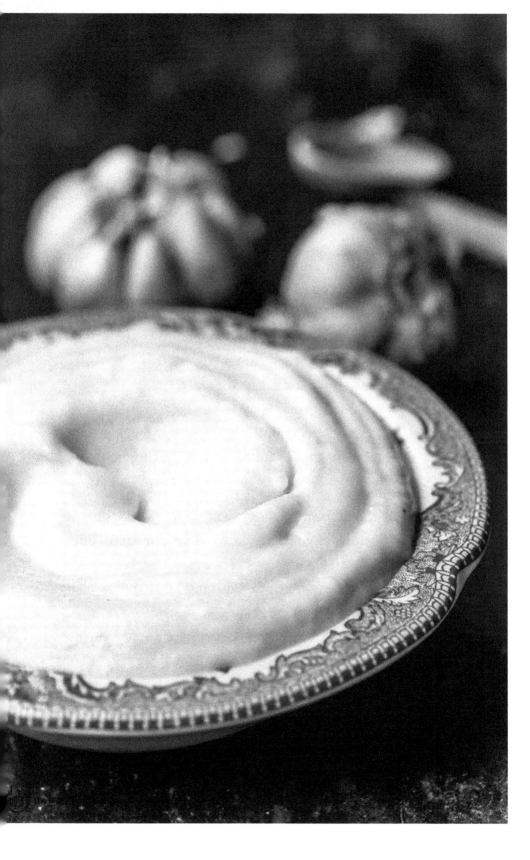

Cannellini Bean Dipping Sauce

Ready in about: 10 minutes

Servings: 12

Per serving: Calories: 123; Fat: 4.5g; Carbs: 15.6g; Protein: 5.6g

Ingredients

- 20 ounces canned cannellini beans, drained
- 2 cloves of garlic, minced
- 4 roasted peppers, sliced
- Sea freshly ground black pepper, to taste
- 1 teaspoon ground cumin
- 1 teaspoon mustard seeds
- 1 teaspoon ground bay leaves
- 6 tablespoons tahini
- 4 tablespoons fresh Italian parsley, chopped

Directions

- Place all the ingredients, except for the parsley, in the bowl of your blender or food processor. Blitz until well blended.
- Transfer the sauce to a serving bowl and garnish with fresh parsley.
- Serve with pita wedges, tortilla chips, or veggie sticks, if desired. Enjoy!
- Enjoy!

SNACKS

Spinach and Mashed Tofu Salad

Ready in about: 40 minutes
Servings: 8
Per Serving: Calories 166 Carbohydrates 5. 5 g Fats 10. 7 g Protein 11. 3 g

Ingredients:
- 28-oz. blocks firm tofu, drained
- 4 cups baby spinach leaves
- 4 tbsps cashew butter
- 1½ tbsps soy sauce
- 1-inch piece ginger, finely chopped
- 1 tsp red miso paste
- 2 tbsps sesame seeds
- 1 tsp organic orange zest
- 1 tsp. nori flakes
- 2 tbsps of water

Directions:
- Use paper towels to absorb any excess water left in the tofu before crumbling both blocks into small pieces.
- In a large bowl, combine the mashed tofu with the spinach leaves.
- Mix the remaining ingredients in another small bowl and, if desired, add the optional water for a more smooth dressing.

- Pour this dressing over the mashed tofu and spinach leaves.
- Transfer the bowl to the fridge and allow the salad to chill for up to one hour. Doing so will guarantee a better flavor. Or, the salad can be served right away. Enjoy!

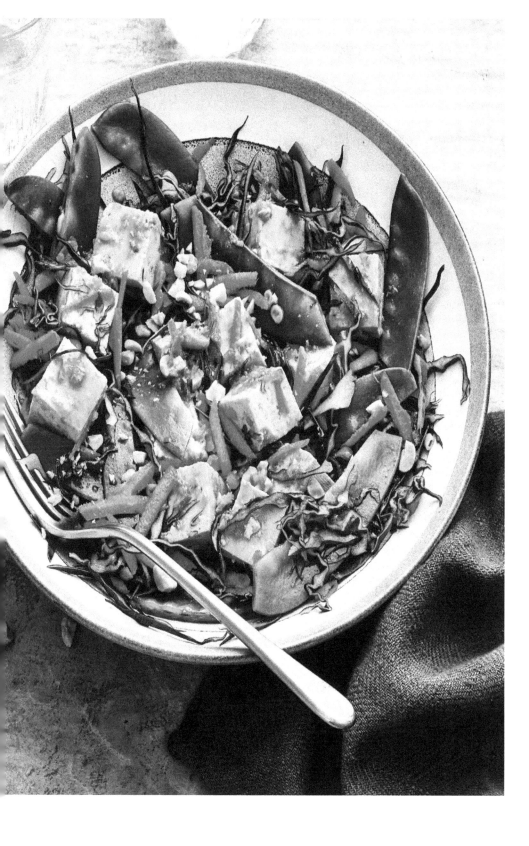

Cucumber Edamame Salad

Preparation Time: 15 minutes |
Servings: 4
Per serving: Calories 409 Carbohydrates 7. 1 g Fats 38.
25 g Protein 7. 6 g

Ingredients:
- 6 tbsps avocado oil
- 2 cups cucumber, sliced into thin rounds
- 1 cup fresh sugar snap peas, sliced or whole
- 1 cup fresh edamame
- ½ cup radish, sliced
- 2 large Hass avocados, peeled, pitted, sliced
- 2 nori sheet, crumbled
- 4 tsps roasted sesame seeds
- 2 tsps salt

Directions:
- Bring a medium-sized pot filled halfway with water to a boil over medium-high heat.
- Add the sugar snaps and cook them for about 2 minutes.
- Take the pot off the heat, drain the excess water, transfer the sugar snaps to a medium-sized bowl, and set them aside for now.
- Fill the pot with water again, add the teaspoon of salt and bring to a boil over medium-high heat.

- Add the edamame to the pot and let them cook for about 6 minutes.
- Take the pot off the heat, drain the excess water, transfer the soybeans to the bowl with sugar snaps, and let them cool down for about 5 minutes.
- Combine all ingredients, except the nori crumbs and roasted sesame seeds, in a medium-sized bowl.
- Carefully stir, using a spoon, until all ingredients are evenly coated in oil.
- Top the salad with nori crumbs and roasted sesame seeds.
- Transfer the bowl to the fridge and allow the salad to cool for at least 30 minutes. Serve chilled and enjoy!

Coconut Veggie Wraps

Preparation Time: 35 minutes

Servings: 5

Per serving: Calories 236 Carbohydrates 23. 6 g Fats 14. 3 g Protein 5. 5 g

Ingredients:

- 3 cups shredded carrots
- 2 red bell peppers, seeded, thinly sliced
- 5 cups of kale
- 2 ripe avocados, thinly sliced
- 2 cups fresh cilantro, chopped
- 10 coconut wraps
- 1/3 cups hummus
- 13 cups green curry paste

Directions:

- Slice, chop, and shred all the vegetables.
- Lay a coconut wrap on a clean flat surface and spread two tablespoons of the hummus and one tablespoon of the green curry paste on top of the end closest to you.
- Place some carrots, bell pepper, kale, and cilantro on the wrap and start rolling it up, starting from the edge closest to you. Roll tightly and fold in the ends.
- Place the wrap, seam down, on a plate to serve.

Cucumber Avocado Sandwich

Preparation Time: 35 minutes

Servings: 4

Ingredients:

- 1 of a large cucumber, peeled, sliced
- ½ teaspoon salt
- 8 slices whole-wheat bread
- 8 ounces goat cheese with or without herbs, at room temperature
- 4 Romaine lettuce leaves
- 2 large avocados, peeled, pitted, sliced
- 3 pinches lemon pepper
- 2 squeeze of lemon juice
- 1 cup alfalfa sprouts

Directions:

- Peel and slice the cucumber thinly. Lay the slices on a plate and sprinkle them with a quarter to a half teaspoon of salt. Let this sit for 10 minutes or until water appears on the plate.
- Place the cucumber slices in a colander and rinse with cold water. Let these drain, then place them on a dry plate and pat dry with a paper towel.
- Spread all slices with goat cheese and place lettuce leaves on the two bottom pieces of bread.
- Layer the cucumber slices and avocado atop the bread.

- Sprinkle one pinch of lemon pepper over each sandwich and drizzle a little lemon juice over the top.
- Top with the alfalfa sprouts and place another piece of bread, goat cheese down, on top.

Carrot Energy Balls

Ready in about: 10 minutes + chilling time
Servings: 8
Per serving: Calories: 495; Fat: 21.1g; Carbs: 58.4g; Protein: 22.1g

Ingredients

- 2 large carrots, grated carrot
- 3 cups old-fashioned oats
- 2 cups raisins
- 2 cups dates, pitied
- 2 cups coconut flakes
- 1/2 teaspoon ground cloves
- 1 teaspoon ground cinnamon

Directions

1. In your food processor, pulse all ingredients until it forms a sticky and uniform mixture.
2. Shape the batter into equal balls.
3. Place in your refrigerator until ready to serve. Bon appétit!

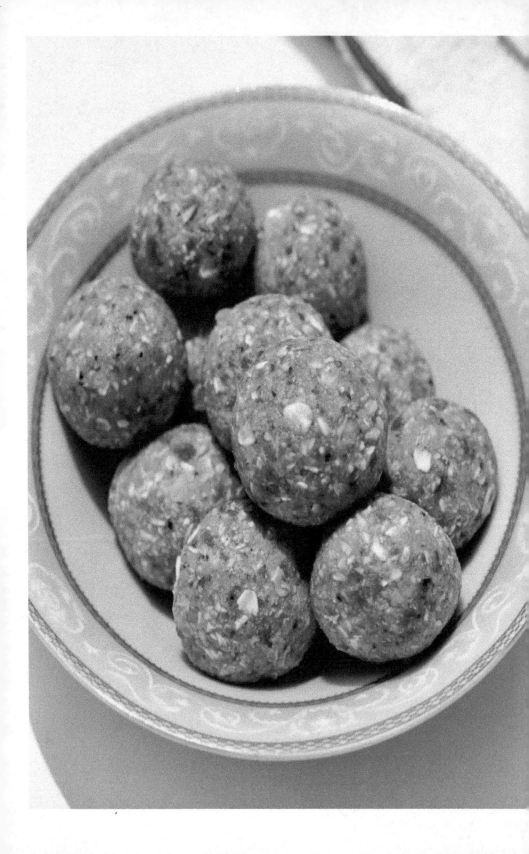

Traditional Lebanese Mutabal

Ready in about: 10 minutes
Servings: 12)
Per serving: Calories: 115; Fat: 7.8g; Carbs: 9.8g; Protein: 2.9g

Ingredients

- 2 pounds eggplant
- 2 onions, chopped
- 2 tablespoons garlic paste
- 8 tablespoons tahini
- 2 tablespoons coconut oil
- 4 tablespoons lemon juice
- 1teaspoon ground coriander
- 1/2 cup ground cloves
- 2 teaspoons red pepper flakes
- 2 teaspoons smoked peppers
- Sea salt and ground black pepper, to taste

Directions

- Roast the eggplant until the skin turns black; peel the eggplant and transfer it to the bowl of your food processor.
- Add in the remaining ingredients. Blend until everything is well incorporated.
- Serve with crostini or pita bread, if desired. Bon appétit!

Indian-Style Roasted Chickpeas

Ready in about: 10 minutes |
Servings: 16)
Per serving: Calories: 223; Fat: 6.4g; Carbs: 32.2g;
Protein: 10.4g

Ingredients

- 4 cups canned chickpeas, drained
- 4 tablespoons olive oil
- 1 teaspoon garlic powder
- 1 teaspoon paprika
- 2 teaspoons curry powder
- 2 teaspoons garam masala
- Sea salt and red pepper, to taste

Directions

- Pat the chickpeas dry using paper towels. Drizzle olive oil over the chickpeas.
- Roast the chickpeas in the preheated oven at 400 degrees F for about 25 minutes, tossing them once or twice.
- Toss your chickpeas with the spices and enjoy!

Onion Rings & Kale Dip

Ready in about: 35 minutes

Servings: 8

Ingredients

- 2 onions, sliced into rings
- 2 tbsps flaxseed meal + 3 tbsps water
- 2 cups almond flour
- 1 cup grated plant-based Parmesan
- 4 tsps garlic powder
- 1 tbsp sweet paprika powder
- 4 oz chopped kale
- 4 tbsps olive oil
- 4 tbsps dried cilantro
- 2 tbsps dried oregano
- Salt and black pepper to taste
- 2 cups tofu mayonnaise
- 8 tbsps coconut cream
- Juice of a lemon

Directions

- Preheat oven to 400 F. In a bowl, mix the flaxseed meal and water and leave the mixture to thicken and fully absorb for 5 minutes. In another bowl, combine almond flour, plant-based Parmesan cheese, half of the garlic powder, sweet paprika, and salt. Line a baking sheet with parchment paper in readiness for the rings. When the vegan "flax egg" is ready, dip in the onion rings one after another and then into the almond flour mixture. Place the rings on the baking sheet and grease them with cooking spray. Bake for 15-20 minutes or until golden brown and crispy. Remove the onion rings into a serving bowl.

- Put kale in a food processor. Add in olive oil, cilantro, oregano, remaining garlic powder, salt, black pepper, tofu mayonnaise, coconut cream, and lemon juice; puree until nice and smooth. Allow the dip to sit for about 10 minutes for the flavors to develop. After, serve the dip with the crispy onion rings.

Sesame Cabbage Sauté

Ready in about: 15 minutes

Servings: 8

Ingredients

- 4 tbsps soy sauce

- 2 tbsps toasted sesame oil
- 2 tbsps hot sauce
- 1 tbsp pure date sugar
- 1 tbsp olive oil
- 2 head green cabbage, shredded
- 4 carrots, julienned
- 6 green onions, thinly sliced
- 4 garlic cloves, minced
- 2 tbsps fresh grated ginger
- Salt and black pepper to taste
- 2 tbsps sesame seeds

Directions

- In a small bowl, mix the soy sauce, sesame oil, hot sauce, and date sugar.

- Heat the olive oil in a large skillet and sauté the cabbage, carrots, green onion, garlic, and ginger until softened, 5 minutes. Mix in the prepared sauce and toss well. Cook for 1 to 2 minutes. Dish the food and garnish it with the sesame seeds.

Herbed Vegetable Traybake

Ready in about: 85 minutes

Servings: 8

Ingredients

- 4 tbsps plant butter
- 2 large onions, diced
- 2 cups celery, diced
- 1 cup carrots, diced
- 1 tsp dried marjoram
- 4 cups chopped cremini mushrooms
- 2 cups vegetable broth
- ½ cup chopped fresh parsley
- 2 whole-grain bread loaf, cubed

Directions

- Melt the butter in a large skillet and sauté onion, celery, mushrooms, and carrots for 5 minutes. Mix in marjoram, salt, and pepper. Pour in the vegetable broth and mix in parsley and bread. Cook until the broth reduces by half, 10 minutes. Pour the mixture into a baking dish and cover with foil.

- Bake in the oven at 375 F for 30 minutes. Uncover and bake further for 30 minutes or until golden brown on top, and the liquid absorbs. Remove the dish from the oven and serve the stuffing.

CONCLUSION

There are a plethora of compelling reasons to make a positive difference and transition to a plant-based diet. A plant-based diet will increase your quality of life by providing you with more energy and stamina, assisting you in losing excess body weight, and perhaps even extending your time in this magnificent world. Too much energy and fossil fuels are lost in the process of obtaining meat and other animal products, shipping them over miles and miles of road, and refining them. You will also be bringing a genuine and important difference to the future of our planet Earth by making the transition.

By switching to rich plant-based meals, we can save the earth and also take care of ourselves. Thank you for taking the time to read this.

CPSIA information can be obtained
at www.ICGtesting.com
Printed in the USA
LVHW021527110521
687091LV00003B/532